Endorsements

Wow! This book is flooded with practical wisdom and raw emotion. Maggie comes alongside those dealing with life-threatening illnesses as a coach and mentor. Filled with truth and transparency, her own struggles and those of others help readers experience a community of friends who have rowed a few miles ahead in this unpredictable exploration.
– Tez Brooks, Writing coach, award-winning author of *Debriefing: Meditations of Hope for Those Who Protect and Serve*

I have walked with Maggie through the ups and downs of her cancer journey and know the perspectives in this book come through hard-fought battles. I'm grateful she's writing this so we can learn from her journey and pass it on to others.
– Andrea Buczynski, Global VP, Campus Crusade for Christ

Everyone can relate to this book, whether it be a personal or loved one's diagnosis. It touches on fear, regret, hope, and faith. The story is shared in a way that moves between the author's personal cancer experience and reflections from others she has crossed paths.
– Karen Selby, registered nurse, author, and Patient Advocate at The Mesothelioma Center

This book will provide you with a triple win: First, you will be moved by Maggie's story. Second, you will be able to understand better the journey of your friends who are walking the same path. And third, you will be better prepared for when you walk through your final days. Last time I checked – none of us are getting out of here alive!
– Bob Tiede, Blogger @ LeadingWithQuestions.com, author of *Great Leaders ASK Questions* and *Now That's a Great Question*.

Raw and honest assessment of life and death's harsh realities combine with poignant yet down-to-earth telling of the author's own cancer battle story to produce a powerful, insightful, and practical guide to navigate the painful journey of terminal illness.
– Kristen Paris, Certified Holistic Health Practitioner, Founder of Powered By Health, and Author of *Beauty From Ashes*.

If you have been given a life-altering diagnosis, you've picked up the right book! Maggie Bruehl understands the path you're walking and the questions you're asking right now—because she's on the same journey herself. In this thoughtfully written and insightful book, Maggie will affirm what you're feeling, share wise perspectives, and encourage you to embrace what matters most at this time in your life.
– Deborah Barr, author of *Strength for the Cancer Journey: 30 Days of Inspiration, Encouragement, and Comfort*

Suspended
Living with Dying

Maggie Bruehl

Suspended
Living with Dying

Copyright © 2023 by Maggie Bruehl
All rights reserved.

No part of this work may be reproduced or transmitted in any form or by any means, electronic or mechanical, including photocopying and recording, or by any information storage or retrieval system, except as may be expressly permitted by U.S. Copyright law. Requests for permission can be addressed to the author, Maggie Bruehl, 5300 South Atlantic Ave 16-503, New Smyrna Beach, FL 32169, or emailed to maggie.bruehl@gmail.com.

ISBN: 979-8-9890658-0-6

Library of Congress Control Number:

This publication is designed to provide accurate and authoritative information in regard to the subject matter covered. It is sold with the understanding that neither the author nor the publisher is engaged in rendering legal, investment, accounting or other professional services. While the publisher and author have used their best efforts in preparing this book, they make no representations or warranties concerning the accuracy or completeness of the contents of this book and specifically disclaim any implied warranties of merchantability or fitness for a particular purpose. The advice and strategies contained herein may not be suitable for your situation. You should consult with a professional when appropriate. Neither the publisher nor the author shall be liable for any loss of profit or any other damages, including but not limited to special, incidental, consequential, personal, or other damages.

For privacy reasons, some names may have been changed.

Book Cover: Sarah Smith (sarahsmithdesigns@gmail.com)

Author Photo: Dawn Roberts

Author's Website: www.maggiebruehl.com

Dedication

I dedicate this book to those living between life and death,
And who are feeling their way through it,
To the best of their ability.

May they find peace in the present moment
As well as for eternity.

Contents

Section 1 – Our Stories 1
Chapter 1 – Beginnings 3
Chapter 2 – Once Upon a Time 7
Chapter 3 – The Unforgettable Day 11
Chapter 4 – Twists and Turns 15
Chapter 5 – Current Reality 19

Section 2 – Caught in the Middle 23
Chapter 6 – The Nature of Death 25
Chapter 7 – The Nature of Hope 29
Chapter 8 – Living in Two Worlds 35
Chapter 9 – Compacted Time 41

Section 3 – Focusing on Today 45
Chapter 10 – Embracing Emotions 47
Chapter 11 – Relationships 53
Chapter 12 – Fighting and Finding 57
Chapter 13 – Finishing Strong 63

For Caregivers 69
In Case You Are Interested 77
Acknowledgments 89
Resources 91
Endnotes 93

SECTION 1

Our Stories

So I'm Not Going to Die[1]

So I'm not going to die,
At least not right now,
Tears of gratefulness.

I had been preparing for the worst,
Thankful for a past,
Confused about my future.

Where do I go from here?
How do I take back my life?
How do I start it up again?

What does my new life look like?
I had a sense of dying,
But not living…

Do I do it as before
Or is it different

Because I am different?
I will never be the same,
Bearing scars of this experience,
Physically and spiritually.

And although they are ugly,
I don't want to lose them
They are real,
A part of who I am.

Life will never be the same,
I know that.

My challenge is
Connecting my life of the past
With the opportunities of the future
Within a life changed forever.

Maggie Bruehl, 2013
Splash: Captured Moments in Time

CHAPTER 1
Beginnings

I HAVE MULTIPLE MYELOMA, an incurable form of cancer. The doctors treat it and knock it back, but it always wins.

Sometimes, I feel as if I am suspended, somewhere between life and death.

We all know that someday we will die. It will be sudden for some, with no opportunity to say a quick goodbye. Others have a disease that will take their life slowly unless an unexpected event intervenes. Whether or not we want to, those with disease have months or years to think about what is coming and to face the question of how to live.

My cancer has been fully active for sixteen years. A precursor was diagnosed ten years previously. My daily reality is that I live with an incurable form of cancer that has never gone into remission.

I can, and sometimes do, become fearful. I pursue medical advice, but I also fight depression and fatalism. Other times, I invest my time in positive ways.

People pick up a book for many different reasons. You may have a disease slowly taking your life. You may have a loved one struggling to understand what is happening in their life. One thing is for sure: you have a reason for picking it up.

I hope the words on these pages will encourage you. I remember years ago reading a book about strong-willed children. After finishing it, I was disappointed it wasn't the "how to" I desperately desired. On the other hand, I was strangely encouraged. Its value was knowing someone else had struggled with child-rearing, made mistakes, and was figuring it out. Someone else *understood*.

This book is similar. It's not meant to be an instruction manual. We are all different people from different backgrounds, dealing with other illnesses in different circumstances.

However, as we think about the future, we do have similarities. We all make decisions daily, intentionally or unintentionally, concerning our lives and how we live them. I am committed to making my decisions in light of who I am, the uniqueness of my disease, and the time I have.

You may think, "I'm not sure I want to read this book. It sounds depressing." It's not a topic I ever wanted to read about, much less write about. But it is where I live each day, and I know other people live similarly suspended.

It can be lonely when we avoid discussing the reality of our disease. Deep down, we hope that it will go away if we don't talk about it. There must be some way to talk about our condition so we can internally accept and process what is happening and invite others into the process as much as they are able. As a result, we will all be richer.

By now, you may have noticed how I matter-of-factly talk about disease and death. It's always been important to me to grasp the reality of the world around me. I can wish my ugly disease away, but it's not leaving.

Let me assure you that I have many emotions that are far from pleasant when I think about dying. I have sought out family, friends, and professional counselors to help along the way.

And although I struggle with emotions, they are my friends. They help me process my past, present, and future. They show me dark, negative thoughts and help me find my way to more positive ones.

One more piece of information about me is that I am a follower of Jesus of Nazareth. I'm sure you will sense it as you read some sections of this book. We all have foundational lenses through which we perceive the world. What you think of life and death is your personal decision, and I respect the freedom each of us has to decide on our worldview. However, my faith can't help but leak into my story, as it is core to my being, just as your values and beliefs are core to yours.

During my journey, I have felt alone. People around me were caring, but they couldn't understand what it is like to know your time may be short. They couldn't feel the pain, emotionally or physically. They didn't sit in a chair, go to work, brush their daughter's hair, or live as if everything was normal, knowing that precious moments were gone with each tick of the clock.

There is strength and comfort in knowing someone else is also struggling, feeling suspended between living and dying.

Reflection:

- Why did you pick up this book?

- What do you hope to get out of it?

CHAPTER 2
Once Upon a Time

LIFE IS NOT A fairy tale, but like all our stories, it starts somewhere.

I grew up a shy little girl in a Czech community on the south side of Chicago, post-WWII. My grandparents lived on the main floor of the flat; my aunt and uncle lived above them while we filled the small, two-bed basement apartment. My parents told us not to play near the garage because of rats, and there were bitter cold winters. My mother was a nurse, acutely aware of her health, a borderline hypochondriac. My father was an accountant, trained during the war, and worked long and hard. Trying not to bother them with my needs, aches, or pains, I found it was safer to be quiet, almost invisible.

Fast forward to when I was 40, married with four children, and moving to a new city. My gynecologist ran a bone density test, announcing I had "stage 3 Osteoporosis — the bones of a 64-year-old woman!" Since my mother had osteoporosis, it wasn't surprising, but his urgency was. He put me on a controversial medication for several months, and when we found out we were moving again, I eventually stopped taking it.

My new gynecologist was as shocked as I was by the previous diagnosis and declared, "You are too young for osteoporosis!" I blushed with the compliment as we began tests to see what was happening. The tests at first revealed nothing, but then she asked me to take one more test by collecting my urine for 24 hours. It sounded strange, but she assured me she didn't think it would show anything. She didn't want to leave any options unexplored.

My husband was out of town when the doctor called with the results. I assumed everything was fine since she called rather than scheduling a visit. However, she told me something did show up in the test, and I needed a specialist. I fumbled for a pencil and paper and began writing as she said, "Call MD Anderson Cancer Center."

I stopped mid-action.

Is this what she was testing for? Cancer? I had no idea. Is that what they treat at a cancer center? Osteoporosis now seemed insignificant as my mind raced uncontrollably.

Sputtering, I wrote down the number and made the appointment. The oncologist got me in almost immediately, which now I know is not a good sign. This time, my husband went with me as moral support.

We were so naïve. The doctor wanted to perform a bone marrow biopsy, and we had no idea what it was. Using only local anesthesia, he drove deep into my hipbone with a hand drill and removed bone marrow with a hypodermic needle. Between the pressure, vibration, and excruciating pain, I almost flew off the table, held only by breathing techniques I learned for Lamaze childbirth classes. Roger almost passed out.

Everything became very real.

With wide eyes and emotions barely below the surface, we met with the doctor to discover the results: Monoclonal Gammopathy. Yes, I made him spell it out and write it down. Just like the name, it was overwhelming. It is a precursor to a bone and blood cancer called multiple myeloma. He assured us it was better to have the precursor because the life expectancy of active multiple myeloma was not good — six to 18 months. But he also explained that it could erupt with no warning at any time. The doctor would test me every three months to be on top of it when it did appear.

How could I go home and tell my children? How can I live my life as if it was normal when it was so far from normal? We could get terrible news in three months, or cancer might never develop. For the moment, we were suspended, not knowing how to continue our lives.

I admit I was in a fog. While going through everyday life as if nothing had happened, we processed new realities. Frantically, I researched multiple myeloma on the internet, finding a few hopeful articles before becoming overwhelmed by obituaries.

I closed the computer. I didn't want to face the future.

• • •

Your disease is lived out in the context of your story, starting with your childhood and basic personality. Life experiences form who we are and how we respond. Like me, you existed before your disease, born in a time and a place. Someone raised you; you grew up in a neighborhood. You laughed; you cried. Your illness does not wipe out everything you are or have been.

But what goes before our disease shapes how we respond to it. My mother and her fear of illness affected me just like your family's attitudes about health and disease affect you. You may have had family members who died with the same disease as you have, causing you to struggle to have hope. Maybe your family didn't discuss their health or death, taboo subjects. Or maybe your family didn't talk about their emotions about anything.

Your story is also financial. You may struggle to pay for treatments or feel guilty for taking time off work since your family depends on your income, your insurance may be maxed, or you may have been denied coverage. Or, you could have good insurance, and finances are not even an issue.

Our relationships are also part of our story. Your disease affects not only you but those around you. Their personalities and values may be different from yours. I remember meeting a woman in the chemo infusion room early in my treatment, both hooked up to machines pumping what would normally be considered poisons into our veins, trying to pass the time as if this was normal. She had moved from

New Jersey to Florida just a year before developing cancer. She had few friends and no children. Her husband hated that she had cancer, that this was happening to them when they finally retired and were supposed to be living "the good life." He wouldn't go into the hospital with her for her infusions, dropping her off at the door. I thought of my husband and the strong support system I felt. Her situation was very different from mine.

Whatever your story is, it is your own story. You can't change the past or how others respond. But we can learn from looking back, understanding ourselves better, and communicating our stories to others.

You and I are unique, with different personalities and circumstances. Your disease is not mine, and your prognosis may not be the same as mine. But with your diagnosis, good health is no longer an assumption. When you were diagnosed, you had to begin to think about life differently. And as you walked toward the future, there may have been more questions than answers.

And there still may be.

But by hearing the beginning of my story, I hope you saw some similarities and, in your mind, began thinking through the context of your story.

It's where we all begin.

Reflection:

- Think about your own story and the context of your disease. How does your background affect your emotional response?

- Think about writing out your reflections. For me, remembering what happened, putting it in words, and seeing it on paper brings reality closer to home.

CHAPTER 3
The Unforgettable Day

I SIGHED WITH RELIEF as time passed and my dreaded cancer didn't develop. Appointments went from every three months to twice a year, and then yearly.

Careers moved quickly as my husband took a global position, and his travel went from national to international. At the same time, my work expanded, and I began international travel with my job. Children grew, married, and started having babies of their own.

Life was periodically interrupted by oncology visits. For the most part, my fear of cancer subsided. My pre-cancerous condition was more of an inconvenience. I confess, I even lost track and skipped a year until I was forced to cancel a trip to Africa at the last minute. The travel center would not give me the yellow fever immunization (a live virus) because of my medical condition, and I was behind in my check-ups.

For the first time since diagnosis, I was furious that I had a condition that limited my freedom.

Later, while traveling in France, I stepped off a curb onto a cobblestone street and jerked my back. Returning home, I saw a chiropractor. In a casual conversation, I mentioned my pre-cancerous condition, and he suggested an MRI to rule everything out.

There it was — the MRI showed a tumor inside my spine, wrapped around my spinal cord. My oncologist saw me quickly and confirmed it was multiple myeloma.

What we feared for ten years was now a reality.

Still incurable, the good news was that treatment for multiple myeloma had progressed. Bone marrow transplants, which had been rare and the last resort, were now done sooner, when patients were stronger, with a better success rate.

During the diagnosis stage, it felt as if everything that could go wrong did go wrong. The tumor biopsy was considered high risk because of its location. It took over a month to schedule surgery. Transferring medical records from hospital to hospital was confusing, and I often had to hand-carry them from doctor to doctor. Once, I even had to retake a brain MRI because of a computer glitch that deleted all test results from one day — the day I had mine, of course!

The biopsy was finally completed, and the doctor confirmed the diagnosis and prescribed treatment. Radiation was not difficult. I relaxed during treatments, giving myself a chance to breathe. I struggled with fatigue but had no major side effects.

Three months later, doctors told me the radiation worked. They were thankful and relieved they had caught it early. I was "good to go" with regular check-ups.

My husband and I celebrated on an Alaskan cruise and bought a new puppy.

Life was good.

• • •

Few of us can forget the day we were told we had a disease that could stop our lives in a heartbeat.

Tracey, newly diagnosed with multiple myeloma, emailed me, "I'm literally in the hospital right now about to have a bone marrow biopsy because they believe I have multiple myeloma. I am 45 with three young children. ☹ I just read your entire blog." Although I had never met Tracy, I could picture her in her little white gown, sitting on the edge of a bed, fingers flying madly across her phone.

A friend of mine, Tip, was an American living overseas. As he remembered the day he was diagnosed with heart disease, he wrote, "My heart attack was from a clot precipitated by playing basketball with two 23-year-old friends. I was taken to a small exam room when about 15 people suddenly appeared, but I felt so awful that the paper gown with no back that it didn't even bother me. What happened next did — two cute nurses started shaving my privates. I was mortified. Before being wheeled into the theater for open-heart surgery, I said goodbye to my treasured wife."

Daily, hundreds are diagnosed with a disease that could kill them. At that moment, their lives are changed. No longer can they assume life but are brought face to face with mortality.

You or your loved one, like me, was diagnosed. You may have been shocked, filled with emotion, or oddly relieved to know there was a name for your symptoms. Like Tracy, you may have sat there alone or been overwhelmed like Tip. As you learned more about your disease, there were emotions, confusion, and decisions.

It was a lot to comprehend.

And then you began your treatment, whether an immediate surgery or waiting for more tests and qualifications. The world did not stand still while you took in everything that was happening. Medical centers lose files. Lab techs miss veins during lab draws (my record was six before they finally struck gold!). Doctors run late, cancel appointments, and sometimes there's conflicting information. It's our life, but it feels like it's spinning out of control.

Plus, we don't just deal with our own emotions but are affected by the feelings of others. I couldn't help but grimace when Kathy casually mentioned, "Oh, my Uncle Joe had multiple myeloma," as she recognized the name of the cancer. As kindly as I could, I asked how Uncle Joe was doing. A little embarrassed, she told me he had died.

In the early days of diagnosis, everything felt simultaneously "fast forward" and "slow speed." Whille the information was overwhelming, life seemed simplified as I understood what was important. Amid the fog, there was clarity. I would just focus on the next thing about to happen.

It takes time to unpack information and emotions, step away from the frantic, and feel a way forward. Nothing is certain. What works for others, medically and personally, may not work for you. Voices, internal and external, can be loud.

It takes courage to follow your path.

Reflection:

- Think about your own story and when you first found out about it. What were your emotions? What were the emotions of others?

- What were the most difficult thoughts you had to deal with? What was most helpful to you?

CHAPTER 4
Twists and Turns

"DO YOU USE ICE or heat on sore muscles?"

Less than four months after hearing the "all clear" from my oncologist, I was feeling great and working out at a local health club when I pulled a muscle in my arm. Since I already had a check-up planned with our family doctor, I casually asked him if I should use heat or cold to ease the pain. Knowing my background, he suggested a quick X-ray, which I did over lunch before returning to his office.

I was unprepared for what happened, as he invited me into his office rather than the exam room. Amid dark walnut bookcases behind his massive desk, he showed me the X-ray. It was clear — cancer had eaten through the humerus bone of my upper right arm. It looked like delicate lace for a one-inch segment where there should have been solid bone.

I was dumbfounded. *Hadn't they just said I was good to go?* I was feeling good, enjoying my freedom. Words totally escaped me. My doctor had already consulted with my oncologist, and appointments were made. Then he asked if he could pray for me. Reality set in.

The oncologist saw me the very next day, and things went into high gear as they found four more tumors in my ribs, collarbone, and shoulder blade. Four days later, I found myself on an operating table, having a metal rod inserted through the center of the bone in my arm. A month after surgery, I began chemo along with steroids and radiation. Two months later, weakened from side effects, I passed out on my bedroom floor, dehydrated, and found myself in the back of an ambulance.

They stabilized me and reduced the chemo while prepping for an autologous stem cell transplant, a type of bone marrow transplant. First, stem cells are harvested from your blood, filtered, and then separated from other types of cells in the blood using a centrifuge. Then doctors kill all the stem cells remaining in your body with chemo, destroying your immunity. My husband still tells the story of seeing the nurses bring the chemo into my hospital room with their yellow industrial gloves to protect themselves, knowing that the very same chemo would flow through his wife's body.

In a race against time, the processed stem cells are inserted back into the bloodstream to regrow before germs challenge the immune system. I developed pneumonia during this process, and I almost died. Slowly, life came back, and my good cells grew. But even with the transplant, my cancer counts never got low enough to qualify as being in "remission."

But at least for a time, I was considered "stable."

• • •

I wish I could say the journey with any disease is a straight path, but it isn't. There are twists and turns, treatments that work and don't work, fears we fight, and hopes we embrace.

My friend Tip wrote, "I got home after two open heart surgeries and being in bed for a solid week. I got into the tub and realized I had no strength to turn on the spigot."

Mandy, a single woman with stage 4 colon cancer, wrote, "If you were to see me or spend time with me, you might be surprised at how normal and full of life I appear. Apart from my belly looking pregnant because of the hernia, the weight I've gained, and the shag carpet of hair under my wig, you wouldn't know I had cancer.

"On the inside, however, I've been grieving and battling fear."

I can relate. I saw my daily life, time, and effort slipping away. Some days, I physically or emotionally couldn't hold even, and some days I went backward.

As much as people around me wanted to lend support, it was hard for them to understand what I was going through. They were not living with my disease. They couldn't creep into my body and feel what I felt, physically or emotionally.

While I was in the most incredible fight of my life, my children became adults, my parents aged and died, and relationships formed while others faded. While I was in the middle of life, I was on the edge of dying. I wanted to be more involved in the world around me, but I didn't know how long or how much I'd be able to contribute. It was hard to grasp what it meant to have a future.

Yet, as time passed, we ended up celebrating days and years. We made plans by the month, not years, around upcoming oncology appointments and lab tests. Every time, we feared the news we might hear.

Suspended, I was trying to grasp the meaning of hope.

Reflection:

- What have been some of your twists and turns medically? Emotionally?

- What have you found to be helpful as circumstances change? What would be helpful in the future?

CHAPTER 5
Current Reality

FOR SEVEN YEARS, "STABLE" was good. My doctor told me that 70 percent of multiple myeloma transplant patients relapse within three years. I enjoyed the time with minimal treatments, made progress in my job, and then retired. We spent time with children and grandchildren. My husband and I even bought a cabin and refurbished it.

My bones were weak, and I broke a wrist and ankle during those years. Healing was complex because of the cancer, requiring two surgeries on the ankle and five on the wrist. But I was determined. Cancer would not take me away from my friends and family.

But the knowledge of my condition was always there. Sometimes I felt guilty. It was difficult to go to funerals for friends. I didn't deserve life any more than they deserved death. We had started a journey together; now they were gone.

While healing from the broken ankle, I went to my oncologist for a regular visit. There had been a steady rise in my numbers, but now cancer indicators were multiplying exponentially. This time I was not as surprised as before. I knew this day was coming, as it always does with multiple myeloma.

There were new chemo medications, so I started on one of them. But soon, doctors had to reduce the dosage as it crashed my immune system. Side effects of fatigue and diarrhea caused me to collapse once again.

Finally, after months of treatment, my body began to respond, the slower-growing healthy cells beating out the faster-growing cancer cells. We got back to that beautiful word, "stable."

Six more years have passed, and I've broken more bones with multiple surgeries. I'm still on this strange journey of being suspended between the land of the living and the land of the dying. Every day has its challenges as well as joy. I live check-up to check-up, waiting for what the oncologist says as he looks at my blood tests, knowing it will set the direction for the next few months or years.

It's hard to describe the tension of living suspended between these two worlds. I wake up each morning glad to be alive, yet very aware that my days may be few.

I know there are others like me who are taking life day by day.

• • •

As I've said before, your story is not my story, and your disease and its progression may be different. You may be at the lowest point of your life, in the middle of treatments, or with treatments no longer available. Or you may be like me, trying to figure out what the word "stable" means.

Karen from NYC recently heard that beautiful word. She's had a rare blood condition threatening her life for over 10 years. She wrote, "At a recent appointment, my doctor looked up and said, "Your labs are nowhere near normal, but you have been stable. So, if you can't be normal, be stable!"

She's claiming it as her new mantra, and we need that little bit of humor, don't we? Wherever you are on your journey, it is helpful to reflect on the ups and downs. Thinking through your own story gives it a sense of reality. The American Society of Clinical Oncology encourages clients to "Take time to reflect. Plan a quiet time to think about your experience and reflect on the changes in your life. Some people prefer to reflect privately, while others decide to share thoughts with family members or friends. You may find comfort through journaling."[2]

All I can say is that our stories don't have neat little endings. We're still on a journey. Some days are tough, while others are enjoyable.

Reflecting on my journey helps me see it objectively and feel it emotionally. It gives me insight into my responses. It helps me know not only what is going on *around* me, but what is happening *inside* me.

For a long time, I didn't want to talk with others who had cancer or other diseases. I hated cancer in my life, and I hated it even more in the lives of others.

But I've found it helpful to talk with people who offer support without judgment or advice or who were going through similar challenges. A few years ago, Cortina, with multiple myeloma in Texas, initiated a Facebook conversation with me. She confessed, "I think I'm more afraid of chemo than I am of death."

She knew that I knew what she was talking about and would listen. She also needed to hear herself say it out loud and know she was heard.

Living in Oregon with multiple myeloma, John wrote, "It is not about just surviving. It's about surviving with grace and poise; it's about surviving with love and compassion for others whose road may be rougher or shorter, and it's about surviving with openness to the miracle of every moment." [3]

It's about being present in the moment because you are still alive. Your story is still being written. Knowing your story affirms the reality of your emotions and perspective. It gives definition and clarity.

It helps us grieve what is lost and celebrate what is good.

Reflection:

- Where are you in your treatment right now? How are you handling it emotionally?

- Do you have safe people in your life who listen? Who are they? Let them know you consider them a trusted friend.

SECTION 2

Caught in the Middle

CHAPTER 6
The Nature of Death

AMERICAN CULTURE AVOIDS DEATH: the topic of death, the smell of funeral homes, the emotions of loss. At the same time, it fascinates us. Religious channels flourish while reality TV glorifies the mysterious ghost hunts. Death from tragedies is a consistent topic on the nightly news, along with pandemics and other health-related topics.

One thing is certain: death comes to us all. If you were born, you will die. Our bridges all lead to another side. Even though it's obvious, we still try to ignore it. Modern science fights it, "saving lives" that eventually will no longer be able to be saved. Our lives are filled with trying to figure out how to avoid death (put on your seat belt, eat your veggies, get your vaccines, etc.) as if we can control death by doing the right things.

Death is a heavy subject. When we have a serious disease, accepting the reality that we might die from it is choosing truth rather than denial. Dr. Tim Keller, with cancer in NYC, put it this way: "Despite my rational, conscious acknowledgment that I would die someday, the shattering reality of a fatal diagnosis provoked a remarkably strong psychological denial of mortality ... I found myself thinking, *What? No! I can't die. That happens to others, but not to me.*"[4]

Valuing Life

Don't get me wrong, accepting disease doesn't mean you rush towards death. Valuing life is a good thing. We give toward humanitarian relief, sending money around the world to help people we have never met. We personally enjoy eating, drinking, and entertainment. We embrace relationships and love.

Every day is a gift. Kara Tippets, a blogger from Colorado Springs, was dying of breast cancer while still loving her husband and four young children. When told there were no other treatments doctors could offer, she blogged, "Each appointment that shortens my days, well, causes me to want to desperately share how very important these small moments are ... that I would give myself time to weep over this bad news, and then I go and capture what life I have left ... that when I come to an end, I will have embraced all the grace, given away all the love, and given to my children and husband what I have kept all these years." [5]

I love her perspective, embracing life and making intentional choices on how to live it. As long as we have breath, there is opportunity.

The Blame Game

When something bad happens, it seems that everyone wants to know the cause. My daughter, upon hearing she was diabetic, immediately asked me, "Does it run in the family? Why did I get it?"

Even if we don't say it out loud, we want to know the cause. Jason, my son-in-law, went to the ER for what was thought to be pneumonia. In just a few hours, doctors were talking about lung cancer. Medical attendants repeatedly asked him, "Do you smoke?" He became so irritated that he asked me to make a sign to go over his bed, "I DON'T SMOKE." He didn't want anyone to feel as if he was to blame, that he had compromised his own health.

Don't misunderstand — there is a benefit in knowing the cause. Research shows that my disease, multiple myeloma, can be inherited. We know asbestos can cause mesothelioma; lead in paint can cause cancer. When we know the "why," we can make changes, no longer using harmful products or testing early, which saves others from risk.

However, it's tempting to play a blame game. We wag our heads about the effects of alcohol or illegal drugs, the environment, our parents, or other factors contributing to disease. If we can't find anyone else, we blame God.

But in our rush to soothe our own needs, we may hurt others. What if Jason had smoked? What if my son inherited multiple myeloma from me? What if you worked around asbestos? Blaming ends with guilt, and guilt doesn't heal.

Simply said: disease is not your fault.

Not a Competition

Another truth: our culture is competitive. We are proud of living long, often taking credit where it may not be due. And even when death is inevitable, we fight, we battle, and some are accused of giving up. Remission is considered a win, while relapse is a loss — all competitive terms. These terms may give courage and energy, but they may also take it away.

My friend Lynn loved her life and lived it fully, even with breast cancer. We were sipping tea on her screened-in back porch when she asked, "When is it okay to stop fighting?" She didn't want family and friends to feel she had quit or given up the battle, yet she felt personally finished. She had peace that she had lived her life well.

Life and death are not a competition we control.

Death is Emotional

And because we value life and love those around us, death is emotional. Everything we know in this world will end. These losses are complicated emotions to embrace, so no wonder we move toward fighting, denial, or withdrawal.

Death is a final separation of relationships. Grieving the sadness of death is normal. There is no way around it.

An insurance nurse called to check in with me and ensure I knew about their services, so she asked, "How are you doing?" I answered her questions and appreciated her input, but then she asked, "Are you sometimes sad?" I knew she was assessing my depression level, but the question felt unfair. Of course, I was sad! Death and disease are not happy subjects.

Differing Perspectives

Living with a disease, especially in our culture, isn't easy. We feel we should put on a happy, courageous face until the end, throwing every dollar into the latest cure. Anything less feels like a failure. But there are other perspectives that embrace the reality of death as well as the value of life.

Facing death may be your last great adventure. You may shudder at the thought but stay with me. I'm sure you've had adventures — marriage, job opportunities, children, living situations. Each one had its challenges. Each one had its lessons.

Why can't facing disease and death be similar? They may not be something to defeat as much as a challenge to address.

In a distorted way, knowing the name of the disease that will probably take my life is a gift. Some go through life unaware of their mortality. My life is more intense and more compact because I know I have limited time. So, I make intentional choices.

I didn't sign up for these health issues, but somehow, I got signed up. While others don't think about death, I live with my reality. My life may be short, while others live without fear of tomorrow.

I look for hope while they assume it.

My challenge is to live suspended in two worlds — living and dying. It's not easy, but it is a way to bring a sense of wholeness, even adventure, into difficult circumstances.

Reflection:

- How do you think culture has affected your feelings about life, death and your disease?

- When you think about making intentional choices, what comes to mind? What are some important things you need to make a choice on and take action?

CHAPTER 7
The Nature of Hope

DEATH IS REAL, BUT let's face it, life is not over.

While the last chapter brought us face-to-face with the reality of death, this chapter focuses on the reality of hope. You have invested your life in people and experiences. They have not dissolved. Even in disease, all is not lost.

It is true that we once thought we had some control over our life, time, and energy. We have less control now, yet we still have some. Hope for tomorrow comes from within us as we live intentionally, making choices in light of circumstances and values.

Hope in Medical Treatments

Medical advances are made daily. When first diagnosed with the precursor for my disease, few treatments were available. Life expectancy was 18 months to two years. Information on the internet was limited, and I quickly came to obituaries. When my multiple myeloma became fully active ten years later, new transplants were available. Now, sixteen years later, new chemotherapy and immunotherapy have been developed. Multiple Myeloma even makes the news when famous people like Tom Brokaw, Geraldine Ferraro, and Steve Scalise developed it.

Doctors don't want to promise miracles and want to give hope.

Pharmaceutical companies tell you their drugs' risks and side effects, limiting their liability, increasing hopes and fears.

My friend and co-worker, Elizabeth, was living with stage four liver cancer. She was an independent, single, working woman, responsible for her own income. Her cancer was found amid an unrelated surgery, making her miss work much longer than expected. When her best option for treatment was another surgery, she couldn't accept it emotionally or financially.

Sitting outside at a Thai restaurant one Florida afternoon, we discussed her options. She had waited over a year since diagnosis to decide about surgery, and it might not be an option if she waited longer. As hard as it was to choose the pain, dependence, and another recovery, she knew that if she wanted a future with her grandchildren, it was something she needed to face.

Nancy was a friend with a recent diagnosis of uterine cancer. Whenever she got a test back that she didn't understand, we would sit in her car reading it together, looking up the words until she understood what it meant. She feared chemo's side effects and decided to go a more "natural" route. I respected and supported her right to choose and encouraged her to do what gave her hope.

One thing is important: whatever treatment you choose, whatever route you take, it should give you hope. Hope may be of a longer life or the assurance that you did everything possible. Hope may also mean stopping treatment.

Whatever hope looks like to you, your decisions are important.

Hope in Emotional Connectedness

Like many emotions, hope can be caught from others. The opposite is also true, as negative emotions like fear can be transferred to you from someone else.

It was the day before we got my final cancer diagnosis, and we were waiting for the biopsy results. Our adult children gathered from the corners of the country to wait with us to hear the report. To make the weekend even more poignant, it was Mother's Day. We sat cross-legged in my husband's home office, eating pizza. In true motherly fashion, I wanted to say something to help them process the words that might be coming. I longed to bind us together as a family so we could emotionally support each other.

My professional background kicked in, and we started talking about their basic personality (introvert, extrovert, etc., from the Myers-Briggs personality assessment). It sparked a conversation about how each one was unique as they dealt with the impending news and helped them anticipate their reactions. It also helped them understand why each would respond differently. I'm glad we shared that moment together and were able to care for each other.

In healthy relationships, each person takes ownership of their emotions. I can talk about my hopes and fears, and others can talk about theirs. We don't have to be the same; in fact, it's good to share and respect our differences. While I need to share my feelings and listen to the emotions of others, I need to remember that their feelings are not mine, and their fears are not mine.

Sadly, some relationships are not healthy. They are not positive, hopeful, or emotionally safe. There may be feelings of judgment, polarizations of right or wrong, and even control issues. Instead of respecting individual choices, some people argue or manipulate others to sway them to their point of view. Instead of bringing people together, relationships are torn apart.

Relationships should be about hope. They remind us of who we are and whom we love. They help us laugh about the past and reminisce about what is good. They allow us to remember what has been accomplished and feel good about the future.

Our lives are not wasted. They are invested in those we love. When you go through a crisis like living with a disease, the value is supporting, listening, respecting, believing in, and hoping for the best.

Hope in Spirituality

There are many religions around the world, and as individuals, we are exposed to different ways to believe. Even those who think there is no

God have a belief system that includes the conclusion that there is no God.

Humans are different from animals, having an awareness that seeks a relationship with God or something bigger than ourselves. There is a desire to touch what is immortal and experience an afterlife. This spirituality gives us a context for pain and pleasure, and good and evil.

I don't pretend to be an expert in religious studies or philosophies. I have my own beliefs and respect the views of others. But I want to make an observation: whatever your belief system, it needs to be strong enough for you to lean into as you deal with life and death. Some believe in heaven or hell, while others believe in soul sleep, reincarnation, or nothingness. Many believe that how we have lived determines our destination, which can be comforting or distressing.

But spirituality is not simply about our final destination. It is also about how we feel about the process of suffering. It may be hard to think about a supreme being who allows suffering and death. Jews talk about *B'Shert*, while Arabs talk about *Kismet*, derived from the Arabic *qisma* (portion or lot). Those of the Christian faith often quote, "God causes all things to work together for good to those who love God."[6] An atheist once wrote, "While our fate is the same, it is the destiny which we can and do control."[7] Whatever our belief system, it should offer comfort.

Our spirituality connects us to a like-minded community. When our faith is weak, others lift us up. They answer questions, receive us as fellow journeyers, and attend to our needs. When we are at the end of hope, they comfort us.

After my diagnosis, I reflected back on what I learned about Christianity and Jesus. I asked more questions about who he claimed to be and what he said about suffering, death, and eternal life. The answers affirmed my faith, both intellectually and emotionally. I remember fumbling through Psalms, highlighting the word "strength" when I was feeling especially weak. I am more convinced than ever of my faith, gaining hope for both my suffering and future.

If your belief system is not working for you, find someone you trust to help you think through what you believe and why. If you have questions, ask them. If answers are not satisfying, ask others. Connect with the part of you that wants answers and desires hope.

And if your current belief system does not give you hope and peace, you might want to find one that does.

Reflection:

- Do you have friends or family who are emotionally safe to express your feelings about your disease and your future? Name them and spend intentional time with them. If not, talk with your doctor about support groups in your area.

- What are your thoughts about spirituality, suffering, and death? Who could encourage you in faith?

CHAPTER 8
Living in Two Worlds

"**HOW DO I LIVE** in two different worlds?"

Mandy looked at me, longing for words of wisdom as we sat with half-eaten lunches. She had stage 4 colon cancer and needed to get her heart and affairs in order. As a single woman, she struggled to balance her treatments, a leadership position at work, and relationships with her extended family, none of whom lived near her.

Figuring out how to live life is challenging for anyone facing disease. It leaves us feeling suspended, somehow caught between different worlds. It's also a challenge for caregivers who know and love those facing disease.

Two Trains, Two Tracks

As Mandy talked, her story resonated with me since my struggles were similar. So, I started to use an analogy.

It wasn't that long ago that my friends and I were blissfully enjoying a ride toward the future, an adventure together on a train into the unknown. We chatted and laughed in anticipation, enjoying the moment. The closest we came to thinking about final destinations was developing bucket lists, a wish list of what we wanted to do before we died. Occasionally, we would cry through a sad movie or hear of a celebrity death, but we chugged on, just grateful it wasn't us.

There were stops the train made. Some were brief hesitations, while others were pure inconveniences. We paused, waiting impatiently as one or two got off the train. We tolerated the stops, hopeful they wouldn't be long and take us off schedule. After all, we had things to do and places to be.

Then, a conductor approached me and told me I had to get off at the next stop and transfer to another train. What a shock! After all, I bought my ticket at the same time as everyone else. They get to continue. It didn't feel fair. We assumed we would be on the same train forever.

The conductor kindly apologized, but there was nothing he could do. He told me that I might be able to transfer back at a future stop, but he wasn't sure. I held on to that hope.

Alone, baggage in hand, I transferred trains. The new passenger car felt empty. Most people were sitting alone or with a close friend. They looked quiet and pale, lost in their own world.

As I found my seat, it felt cold and hard, unfamiliar. The engine began to cough and chug as it took me away. I looked out the window, longing to be with my friends on the first train. Sometimes we ran on parallel tracks or stopped at stations, close enough to see each other, wave, or yell out the windows. They assured me my train would stop soon and we'd all be back together again. As time went by, I was less sure.

The conductor was compassionate. He told me about stops along the way, but it all seemed confusing. I wanted to be with my friends, but they were headed elsewhere. They couldn't envision where I was going. Neither could I.

Circumstances didn't change, so I started to relax in my seat, moving my suitcase around to be more comfortable, and even finding ways to entertain myself. I exchanged shy smiles with those in my car. A few wanted to talk. We shared similarities in our stories. And although we missed our old trains, we were learning to accept our new journey.

The Power of Choice

Mandy loved the train illustration and knew exactly what I was talking about. She had gone from hospital treatments to the office, all in one day. She had to work through her own fears about death while trying to assure others. She straightened her wig, put on her make-up, and tried to look normal when she knew life was anything but.

I shared with her that cancer made me live life more intentionally. Instead of life happening to me, I was determined to make as many choices as possible to live out my vision and purpose. We don't think about how the little moments in life add up, determining our future. While we want to do good things in our lifetime, sometimes we don't take advantage of opportunities and squander what we have. When we let life happen to us, we become victims.

Instead, we can set priorities with as much strength as we have. For example, when diagnosed, I need to make my health a priority. While others prioritized their weight and nutrition because of their looks, for me, extra weight put stress on my bones, causing fractures.

Relationships have always been a priority for me. As energy became an issue, my circle of friends and family members became smaller, with deeper roots. Together, we drew the courage to go into parts of our lives we had been afraid to explore. Our relationships were honest, without pretext, because there just wasn't time or energy not to be.

How I did my job has also changed, as I valued the flexibility to reduce stress and physical exertion. I quit traveling internationally and began co-leading projects so that the project wouldn't be jeopardized if my health suddenly took a turn. Coaching young leaders and transferring what I have learned became an important part of my new job description.

Managing my energy was essential, especially in how it affected my relationships. Sometimes I pushed myself, using up my strength until I was no longer pleasant to be around. By carefully choosing my activities, I saved energy for those I valued the most.

Mandy and I discussed schedules — how do you make plans when you don't know how you will feel? The temptation is to overextend, thinking of what we can accomplish on a good day and hoping to repeat it the next day. We're afraid that if we limit our expectations to what we can do on a bad day, our negative thinking will somehow cause the next day not to go well. And if it's a good day, will we be bored with nothing to do? Or worse yet, will someone think we are lazy?

So far, I haven't lacked things to do when feeling better than expected. Sometimes I just rest up for the next treatment. I try not to ramp up my schedule until I've felt better for several weeks because different treatments have different fatigue factors. And so far, no one has thought I was lazy!

I would rather people be surprised by what I've accomplished than disappointed because of unfulfilled commitments.

Self-forgiveness and Letting Go

And then there is self-forgiveness, a helpful skill for anyone dealing with disease. Even those who don't have a disease need a dose of it!

We didn't ask for a train transfer. We didn't plan on having this disease. Deep down, most of us feel we deserve a full life. But slowly it sinks in, and by accepting our new route, we get a little more comfortable in our seats. The routine becomes part of our new reality.

I just can't do all that I used to do. The energy, the health, is not there. When I can't finish projects, am late on an assignment, or forget to call a friend, I need to forgive myself and ask for forgiveness. Usually, others give it far more freely than I give it to myself.

This is a time to make ourselves a priority. We give to others for much of our lives, but if we want more time in the future, we must make ourselves a priority. At the beginning of each week, before I put anything else in, I schedule rest and exercise. I don't always realize my good intentions, but I try to prioritize them.

Something else, here is a time to let go of things you can't change. We all want to look and feel normal, but sometimes that's impossible. We want to accomplish great and small things, but sometimes that's impossible. We want to love and give to others, but sometimes that's impossible.

We may need to let go of some relationships. Some people are stuck in their ways, and as much as we want peaceful relationships, things won't change. Pursuing the relationship may take too much initiative, especially when struggling with limited time and energy.

At the end of our discussion, Mandy took a deep breath as she thought more about the trains. A few days later, she blogged her own thoughts on how she is learning, "to live on two tracks: fully engaged with this earthly existence while planning and preparing as if time is short. I can be going throughout my day or week, making my list of things to do, places to go, and people I want to see. In a matter of seconds, when a side effect takes over, or the doctor calls with bad news, I switch over to the other track, doing only the necessary and extremely important. I might buy new bathroom towels one day, thinking I'll be around for a while. The next moment, I'm giving away precious possessions to people I love. Maggie has shown me grace and permission to live in this place, numbering days and living with a heart of wisdom."

Reflection:

- How do you resonate with the illustration of the two trains? What do you miss most about the first train?

- Now that you are on the second train, what intentional decisions can you make to ease the journey?

CHAPTER 9
Compacted Time

THE MORNING GREETS ME with the scars and bruises from different medical procedures. Waking up to a yellow-striped chemo pill each day is a not-so-subtle reminder that my life is far from ordinary, no matter how good I may feel. My day starts differently than the person in the next office cubicle, driving down the road next to me, or dropping off their child at school.

And if we aren't careful, dealing with a disease can lead to anxiety and depression. We live with fears others can only imagine. They have the luxury of ignoring death while we live with daily realities. It's a heavy weight that's hard to balance.

But if we don't balance the reality of dying with living life to the fullest, disease declares victory over precious time and opportunities. Rather than be helplessly suspended, we need to choose to live intentionally in their world even if they cannot come into ours.

Intentional Living

What others take for granted is no longer ours: health, happiness, holding our children, laughing with friends. Without realizing it, they wake each morning to view a future much different from ours. They may dread aspects of the day or challenges of the future. They may not like their boss or want to move to Montana, but they can have a perspective of time and ability that gives them power over circumstances. The question hovers over the whirlwind of the morning, *what will they do with that power?*

Last night I was on a phone call with a support group of Mesothelioma patients. Usually, the group chats about treatments and clinical trials and is upbeat about their options. Patricia, newly diagnosed, was on the call. She listened to the banter for about an hour and then asked, "What keeps you guys going?"

Silence.

The mood turned somber. Terry from Tennessee broke the ice, "We all know this thing is terminal. Maybe it's just my stubbornness that keeps me going."[8] Others cited medical hope, meditation and personal faith, the survival instinct, and focusing on personal goals. But the heaviness of the future's reality is undeniable.

Even though we live with a disease, we still have choices. We can succumb to denial, fear, or depression. We can keep our feelings to ourselves, pretending to be on the same train as all our friends and family. We can "go with the flow," knowing our stream will shortly break off and head in a different direction.

Depression takes a lot of energy. I know because I've been there. It's exhausting. I needed help to escape the cycle of negative thinking and make different choices.

But as much as I feel powerless in my circumstances, I am not. Life has become more compact, but that also means my power, influence, and time have more impact.

My story, which includes what I am going through, catches the attention of others. They are interested in my health, of course, but they care even more about how I deal with the reality of death because they know that someday they may be in my place. Some have even said I have an "advantage," being able to feel the endpoint of life.

As Rhonda, my friend with breast cancer, asked herself, "What choices am I making today that show I understand how precious time is?"

Living a Compressed Life

Somewhere in the process, I realized I still had choices, not just in determining medical treatments, but in how I responded personally to the diagnosis. I could compact pain and grief into these final years or moments, or I could compact influence, love, and hope. Either way, I was going to make an impact on those around me.

I've been around death more times than I would have liked these last few years. I've seen ones that went well with a family together, holding hands, praying, and singing. And I've also been where it did not go as well — individuals in the same room but not connected to each other or the one dying. I've heard bitter statements of what could have been or longing for what wasn't said.

A friend, Terry, blogged about her mother's death: "In my memories, my parents fought all through my childhood … for almost 30 years they have lived in the same city, but never saw each other. We arranged every holiday and family event around which parent we would visit or which one of them would be invited to attend. It could never be both at the same time. They will never know how many hours of exhaustive planning, debate, maneuvering, and heart anguish accompanied each special occasion through the years.

"This Thanksgiving, something amazing happened. My parents agreed for the first time to give thanks together. The death of a spouse, terminal cancer, and years passing finally cleared the way for reconciliation, acceptance, forgiveness, and peace. It was a powerful, healing moment for everyone, even the grandchildren, to watch my parents greet each other at the front door." [9]

Spoken or unspoken, we fear the end of life. We know it will involve pain and separation, things we avoid. We know death is inevitable. We spend years educating ourselves on how to live, succeed, and overcome challenges, but we have few models of how to die. It touches places so deep that we fear what it will be like.

Maybe it is my stubbornness, but I refuse to waste any of this compact life. A few moments ago, I stopped in the middle of writing, reaching up to intentionally give my 6'2" son a hug. With tears in my eyes, I told him that although he is very much a man and we don't often talk about emotions, I would always love him as my little boy. He knew what I was saying. With a broken voice, he responded, "You can love me like a little boy any time you want."

Words are powerful. Time is short. Life is compact. We all have choices on how to use our power in light of our time, but this is sure: it *will* have an impact.

Reflection:

- Why do you hesitate to discuss your journey and feelings about your disease? What would help you to overcome your hesitations?

- What is an intentional choice you could make that would move you in the direction you want to go? What first step could you take?

SECTION 3
Focusing on Today

CHAPTER 10
Embracing Emotions

LIVING WITH A DISEASE is not only a suspension in our lives, but it can also be an emotional roller-coaster. Every test, doctor's appointment, side effect, pain, and even conversation with friends evokes emotions that squirm out of control. As much as we try to lasso them, they still escape.

There is the initial shock of the diagnosis and confusion that comes from trying to make sense of it all. We badger ourselves into figuring out where the disease originated and, "Why me?" While others seem to lead charmed lives, between the fatigue and pain we may be experiencing, anger and jealousy raise their ugly heads.

The Spiral

Disease threatens our sense of independence, something we intensely value and develop from childhood. For example, my son-in-law, Jason, had a physical therapy appointment after an industrial accident that mangled his ankle. His wife could not drive him and asked me to do it. However, the thought of depending on his mother-in-law to drive him around town was more than this 20-something-year-old could bear — he ended up canceling!

Jason's ankle did heal over time, but it's even more challenging when you have a disease leading to death, knowing you will become more dependent on others as time passes. There is the embarrassment that comes with physical challenges, like needing a walker, wheelchair, or help up a curb. Chemo brain and confusion are also embarrassing. My most significant side effect from medication is diarrhea, and you can imagine how hard that can be to manage!

We struggle to control our schedules, relationships, lives, and self-image. Kate blogged, "Cancer has kicked down the walls of my life. I cannot be certain I will walk my son to his elementary school or subject his love interests to cheerful scrutiny. I struggle to buy books for academic projects I fear I can't finish to prepare for a perfect job I may be unable to keep. Cancer requires me to stumble around in the debris of dreams I thought I was entitled to and plans I didn't realize I had made."[10]

And in trying to control our lives physically, we sometimes try to control others relationally. We don't want to listen about their lives, the things they can do while we can't, the foods they eat, or the plans they make that we won't share. We don't want to tell them our emotions or hear theirs. We want to protect ourselves from any more feelings, pulling the covers over our heads.

But loneliness only deepens depression. Without an outlet, our emotions turn inward, eating up more of our strength than they deserve. We can end up in a cycle that does not produce relief.

Justin, with chronic myeloid leukemia from Texas, wrote, "My diagnosis represented a dark place. It symbolized heartache, frustration, and futility, emotions that don't constitute a life worth embracing. The thought of filtering out so many negative emotions was overwhelming. I tried to fix the uncontrollable instead of focusing on what I could control."

Reversing Direction

"So, when the certainty of your mortality and death finally breaks through, is there a way to face it without debilitating fear?" Dr. Tim Keller asked in the last year of his life.[11]

It's not easy to envision a future, much less a positive one, and

I'm not going to appease you with pat answers. When I get caught in the spiral, it's a signal that I need to talk to someone to interrupt the negative thoughts rolling around in my head. It may be a professional or a trusted friend who will listen and value my emotions without putting their emotions on me.

Talking with someone confirms the reality of what I am experiencing, physically and emotionally. It brings what is inside me into the light of day. When it becomes a shared audible, it becomes a shared experience. The other person can confirm what is happening to me and how my feelings are reasonable, considering the circumstances. That affirmation is life-giving.

It also stops the spiraling and gives me a new place to start. The person probably has some thoughts of their own that are different from mine, giving me other perspectives to consider when I am alone. A friend of mine, Sue, dealing with Hodgkin's Disease when I was going through my transplant, offered some simple advice: "One thing that I found important was to not focus on cancer. I know it seems all-consuming right now but try to find other things that challenge you so that the cancer is a 'by the way' thing as much as possible. So, what I want to hear is a little of what delights you as you go about your week."

What delights me? That question felt so far from anything I was experiencing! But the more I thought about it, the more things came to mind. First, they were simple, like realizing it was time for another pain pill. Then it grew into a desire for caramel macchiato ice cream or my husband's kiss on my forehead. When I was more mobile, it was planning a trip or finding seashells on the beach. The "delights" changed as my physical and emotional levels changed, but I still find it an intriguing thought.

A cancer website encourages us to "celebrate milestones." How we celebrate will vary with our personalities and disease, but noting when things have changed and how they have changed gets us out of the mundane "every day is the same; it will never change" kind of thinking.[12] Milestones may be toward health or death, but just acknowledging them gives us the feeling of movement. Talking with others about them provides us with a sense of reality.

Another blog gave me a couple of interesting thoughts. It connected purpose with growth in empathy: "Since my personal journey with cancer began, I increasingly felt that part of my purpose in life was to be an encouragement to others. I developed empathy for those who are also on the journey ... A waiting room was no longer a necessary evil; it was an opportunity to appreciate my journey and how far I had come. Being around others with similar illnesses is a unique opportunity to identify with patients fighting the same battles and sharing the same hope. We're all in it together, tied by a common bond, asked to endure a diagnosis we would have otherwise said we couldn't handle." [13]

I had a choice as I sat in waiting rooms or chemo units. I could feel sorry for myself and think about all I wanted to be doing instead of being there, or I could develop empathy for those around me. I noticed a new girl in her late 20s as she sat alone in the corner, looking nervously at her papers in a manilla folder. There was an elderly African-American man trying to reassure his wife that everything was going to be OK, although their faces showed they both knew differently. Although an introvert by nature, my cancer gave me new boldness to say something to each of them, letting them know a little of my story and how I have hope. It also gave me a renewed purpose.

Obviously, your purpose may be different from mine. Because of your disease, you have a unique understanding of life. I would encourage you to use your empathy to reach out to others.

Our spiritual faith also affects our emotions. If you believe in a loving God, even if he doesn't feel so loving while you are suffering, there should be comfort in your faith. If you believe in an afterlife or even nothingness, that should be comforting. There will be an end to your direction, and your faith should help you along the way.

What will we do with the feelings we have along the journey? Our emotions can be our friends, helping us know the unconscious thoughts that motivate choices. And even if we ignore our emotions, they don't go away. In fact, they control us more, becoming intense as they dive deep inside. If we acknowledge them, they become quieter, as if they are being listened to.

Listening and talking about emotions can help you make choices for your future, not *despite* your emotions but *inspired by* your emotions.

Justin, whom I mentioned earlier, wrote this: "After sitting in a cold, lonely apartment that winter, I made the decision to embrace my illness … I made the commitment to understand complex emotions, grow as a human being, and push myself through the realities."

That choice is up to you. You can sit in the emotions and spiral down, or reverse the direction with the strength that you have.

How you handle your emotions is one of the few things you can still control.

Reflection:

- Where are you along the spiral of emotions related to your disease? What can you do to reverse the direction?

- What is something that delights you? Make it your goal to find something today that makes you smile.

CHAPTER 11
Relationships

I'LL NEVER FORGET THE ashen look on Roger's face as we left the doctor's office after they did my first bone marrow biopsy. It took days for him to talk about how helpless he felt as the doctor bore into my hip with the drill. That was when I realized that cancer was not just happening to me but was also affecting others around me.

I have been fortunate to have a husband walking alongside me, but whatever your situation, know that it impacts those around you. There is a woman in Michigan with dementia who has a saint of a neighbor and walks her back to the house when she gets confused at the mailbox. My single friend, Pam, leaned on neighbors and friends when she was fading. Our children and co-workers are affected. We all have made a mark on this world, and others see that mark.

Managing the Emotions of Others

We do not exist alone; we are in a context. And just as we have our emotions, those around us have their emotions. A challenge in relationships is keeping boundaries, with each person responsible for their own actions and emotions.

Confusing emotions go off during a conversation. As we listen to others and begin to have our own emotions about what they are saying, we are tempted to project onto them what we feel. For example, if you tell me your daughter is moving to Idaho, I might think you are sad because you will miss her. After all, I would be sad if my daughter moved to Idaho. But you might be relieved because of the pressure you felt to care for her little children. If I projected my sad feelings on you, you might feel guilty that you didn't feel sad.

When I talk about my incurable cancer, some people get overwhelmed. They imagine the fear they would feel if they had received a diagnosis as dire as mine. It would be easy for me to lean into their fears, feeling that I should be more fearful.

Projection goes beyond empathy, which is the ability to understand and share the feelings of someone else. It assumes the other person has certain feelings because we have them. And if we have them and they don't, then something must be wrong with them or us.

See how things get intertwined and distorted? A person can start with one feeling and end up with another. Listen carefully when talking with others, and make sure they understand what you are feeling and why. If they don't understand, don't be shy about expressing yourself. Remember that they are still on the other train (Chapter 8) and won't naturally understand your journey because they are not experiencing it.

Bottom line: everyone needs to own their emotions. I guarantee you I have enough emotions, and you have enough, and we don't need to be catching them from each other. So, when I see a person's feelings on their face when I tell them about my cancer, I put a virtual fence or boundary around my feelings so that theirs can't come in. They need to own their feelings just as I'm responsible for mine.

That leads me to discuss what it means to have safe relationships. We all need safe people in our lives, whether we have an illness or not, people who respect us for who we are and don't try to project or transfer their feelings onto us. We need people who keep our confidence and treasure our opinions. We don't need people who compete with us, correct us, or try to sell us their perspectives. I encourage you to identify safe people you can relate to and encourage those relationships.

Helping others

And visa-versa, we can become safe people to others, careful not to project our emotions onto them. They may be feeling the loss of their relationship with you as their friend, husband, mother, etc. Emotions need to be heard, and sometimes you are the best person to hear them. If they need to confess shortcomings you have forgotten years ago, listen and don't brush them away. These feelings need to be expressed, just as you need to express yours.

As they realize you are not trying to influence their emotions, they can relax in who they are along with who you are. You will begin to journey together from unique perspectives. Together you can love, respect, and support each other during difficult times.

But not everyone travels at the same speed in accepting the realities of your disease. Some will not understand or will be in denial longer. We don't want to force reality on them but encourage them to embrace reality as much as possible. There is kindness in telling a child that "Mommy is sick" rather than "Mommy is going to die." In the same way, we can meet others where they are in the journey, encouraging them toward reality.

Time has a way of helping. We may be painfully aware that time is slipping by, but others may not.

Counseling and Support Groups

Relationships are critical in life as well as when we face death, and few of us are truly prepared for the pain and grief.

Counseling can be especially beneficial. Your physician's office should be able to connect you to licensed counselors who will listen and help you understand the validity of your feelings during this complex journey. They can also help you discern what others are feeling and how best to respond.

Personally, I have found support groups helpful as I listen to a variety of experiences from different perspectives and personalities. Coming away from the group, I know I am not alone. I usually have new ideas to consider and ways of problem-solving. And if nothing else, I know others are working through similar situations.

Rhonda, with breast cancer, said it this way, "My support group has my heart as we journey together... My self-protective side says, 'Don't put yourself through any more grief. Drop out.' But my heart says that these folks are important to me, and celebrating the joys and triumphs together is definitely worth it."

Caregivers

Let's not forget the most important relationship of the journey, your caregiver, the person who has been the closest to you throughout your illness. They need you to communicate with them not only your needs but your appreciation. They will not do everything perfectly, just like none of us does everything perfectly. But they are sacrificing to be with you during the most challenging part of your life. It could be easy for you to blame them for things that are not their fault while in your own pain and need. So, as you are able, give them grace and understanding.

Their job can be overwhelming. On top of caring for you, they still have all the other elements of their life. Listen to and help them as much as possible. My friend, Sue, with leukemia, wrote, "Paul is overwhelmed by caring for me, his folks, the kids, the house, etc., but your e-mail prompted a great conversation, and we are going to change some things around here, so he can get back to the things he needs to be doing."

Oliver Sacks, a blogger summed it all up with, "I cannot pretend I am without fear. But my predominant feeling is one of gratitude. I have loved and been loved; I have been given much, and I have given something in return."[14]

Reflection:

- What emotions have others thought you should have? How are they different from your own?

- What is your next step in improving your relationships?

CHAPTER 12
Fighting and Finding

BRAVE...WHAT DOES IT MEAN to be brave?

That was the opening line on a blog I posted several years ago, and to this date, it is the most commented-on post. Some comments were from people in the same place in life, wanting to be brave themselves. Others were looking in from the outside, wondering how I was handling it, asking themselves, *what would I do if I were in her place?*

But you really don't know until you are there how you will respond. You've read online articles, listened to doctors, heard the stories about the end of patients with your disease, and know some of what to expect.

But how will *you* handle it? That's still an unanswered question.

Fighting Disease

The response to fear is "flight or fight," and since we can't flee our own bodies, we choose to fight the enemy that tries to take it away. We research and consult with different doctors. It seems like there is always a new medication that may or may not promise success or relief. We learn as much as we can to make the most informed decisions, but I must admit, sometimes I give up in sheer exhaustion.

One helpful hint I've passed on to others is to have someone go with me to doctor's appointments. Maybe it's my chemo brain, or perhaps it's just the complexity of cancer, but sometimes when the doctor is talking, what he says gets muddled in the clinical terms and legal language. He may be giving me alternatives, not trying to sway me one way or the other, which makes it hard to feel the pros and cons. His suggestions are based on scientific results but can't tell me if the treatment fits my values, lifestyle, circumstances, or expectations.

On the way home from the appointment, it's helpful to discuss with the partner what was said and how we understood it. Sometimes the other person hears information I haven't caught. There may be a feeling they felt during the appointment, a fact my mind raced over, or a different perspective.

A few years ago, a doctor recommended a procedure that was costly in time, money, and pain. My husband and I tried to reason through it, but we found ourselves spinning in circles, so I asked several of my children for their thoughts. My son patiently listened and then offered, "Why wouldn't you do it if it makes the time you have left less painful?" The simplicity of his response and the perspective of his question left me speechless, but the direction was clear. To this day, I don't regret that procedure.

And then there are times when there are no more medications, or you decide you no longer want to go through treatment. Ethan, a blogger with cancer, made that difficult decision and posted, "I believe there is a point where the quality of life provided does not justify additional efforts to extend life." [15]

We each put our options through a grid of what we value most to come to a conclusion. One friend of mine refused chemo because she was afraid of side effects more than she feared death. Another friend wanted to pursue every reasonable option until there were no more. Still another wanted to be around every moment of her children's lives, just to see another coloring page come home from school or smell a freshly picked flower.

I can't forget the simplicity of the statement Laurie Becklund wrote in her blog: "Promise me that you'll never say I died after 'fighting a courageous battle,' suggesting that our fight was ever fair." [16]

Our illness never feels fair as we look at all the healthy people in this world, no matter how hard we fight.

Finding Peace

Finally, we know in our hearts the battle is over. I've seen it several times — options for treatment are exhausted, the body can no longer fight, and physicians talk about hospice or palliative care. The focus shifts from active treatment to wrapping up life.

Those are hard words to hear.

When that time comes, it's important to find peace. You have fought the fight; now it's time to let go. We don't want to, but it has been inevitable that this day would come. It's not losing a battle but accepting the reality of life. There is grief in letting go of all we have known.

Mandy, whom I have mentioned before, approached this season with as much energy as she could muster and called it her "end game plan." She tried to envision her last weeks of life and where she wanted to spend them. She had lots of friends, and since her family was having difficulty between themselves, she picked a friend she felt could handle the responsibilities and emotions of her final days. She clearly communicated her wishes to her family and included them in the burial, but she preferred time with those she felt emotionally and spiritually close. As hard as it was, her passing went well.

Like Mandy, we can simplify and, as much as possible, control our end of life. Kristin, a single woman in her 50's, knew her passing would most affect her mother. Leaving her friends, she stayed with her mother several states away. It was one last gift she could give her, to be with her at the end.

There are other aspects of the end of our life we can control. While it's hard to imagine, others are often relieved when we realistically talk to them about it, express our opinions, and take responsibility for as much as possible. For example, leaving an updated DNR is essential, so others don't have to make heart-wrenching decisions. I remember a conversation in a hospital hallway when there was no

DNR. The state and doctors began making very personal decisions regarding the life of a dear friend that I knew in my heart she would not want to be made.

We also have some control over how we will be remembered. Sometimes, there is a marking of our lives after our passing, like a funeral or memorial service. It's helpful for planners to know our wishes concerning it. This could include favorite readings or scripture, especially meaningful songs, and people we would like to speak. I chuckle even now, remembering our son-in-law's memorial service and the photo montage backed by a country tune and the line, "I got my toes in the water, ass in the sand." The minister commented that it was a first at that church, but it was also so "Jason," fitting his personality to a tee.

Having an updated will may also seem like a formality, but it is very important. It shows how you want your life work, possessions, and loved ones treated. All that is left on earth converges into a single document. I've seen several situations where there was not a will, leaving the family and government trying to figure out what happens to possessions that were once so personal and valued. With so many convenient computer programs like Quicken Will and internet services, it's not difficult or expensive.

Another detail is cremation or burial and the final resting place. I've seen families split over these decisions, adding to their pain while already grieving a loss. Anything you can decide in advance will give those you love peace. It is a gift.

Don't be afraid to approach these subjects with those close to you. You may not want to make them sad, but they are sad already, knowing an end is coming. It will give you peace to communicate these things before they are needed, before everyone is overwhelmed, and they won't have to make decisions in a vacuum after you are gone.

And don't feel like you are being too bossy and directing what others must or must not do — they can change the plan as necessary, and you won't be there to know the difference!

Reflection:

- What do you need to do as you "fight" your illness? Are there changes you need to make?

- What do you think will help you find peace when the time comes? What can you do to help others find peace?

CHAPTER 13
Finishing Strong

BUT OUR JOURNEYS ARE not over yet, which is why I am writing, and you are reading. What we are going through is different from people who assume good health. We don't know how our journey will end or when it will end, but we know it will end. In the meantime, we're trying to figure out how to make the time we have count the most.

One thing that makes it difficult is the feeling of suspension, of transition from one place to another. We were once a healthy, younger version of ourselves. When we got the diagnosis, we transitioned into someone wearing a new label, learning new ways of living, and facing new challenges. As our health went up and down, our labels changed, creating hope, and dealing with disappointments. For some of us, it's been a long ride, and while adjustments have been challenging, we've made them and are glad for the extra time. For others, it has been shorter.

It's good to know we are not alone. Others know what it feels like to go through these challenges, going to doctor's appointments, endless tests, reactions to medication, special diets, and deliberate exercise. Even as I write this, I'm dealing with diarrhea, and canceling my plans for dinner. I seem to get it after taking my chemo drug on my "three weeks on, 1 week off" schedule. But I know to some, this would be mild compared to what you suffer. For others, it's not the physical challenges but the emotional ones, fearing a pick-up basketball with grandkids might end up in a heart attack or the discipline of not eating your daughter's wedding cake because of your diabetes. You never know what will happen as you live with your disease.

While we all die, some are just sooner than others. Some of us live longer, but with a disease that will someday take our lives. It gives us time to think, to count days, months, even years. But it also makes us feel suspended somewhere between life and death.

I've lived long enough to have "survivor's guilt." Like many other feelings, it leaves you caught between the joy of surviving and the guilt of surviving. I've seen others pass who were younger, healthier, wiser, and even better people than myself and wondered, *why me?*

I may never know the answer, but for whatever reason, I am surviving. I am still here and committed to taking advantage of every moment with intentional living. I can't help but believe that one of the reasons I am still alive is to write this book and encourage others on the journey.

It's Not Easy

We've talked a lot about how living with a long-term disease has felt to me. You have heard my story, and I wish I could sit down with you and listen to yours. You may be anywhere along the spectrum of life, but the truth is, someday, you will be at the end of it.

I remember when Mandy wrote, "It's truly a roller coaster on most days. Yesterday I was just weary and 'over it.' I am so over being sick, so over looking hideous, so over my limitations. I also feel a sense of grief, grieving the days gone by and the loss of relationships, abilities, roles, a voice, and a purpose." My heart ached for her, knowing that one day, I would be in the same place.

Ethan posted, "I felt like my body was shutting down. I felt like I was close to death. And, truth be told, I was kind of looking forward to dying. I was tired of the constant struggle, tired of my life being dominated by my medical condition, and tired of feeling sick all the time." [17]

There is a point when our purpose for the future, our thinking, shifts from "someday" to "that day." We know the day is coming when things will not get better. It's a gracious warning to get our thoughts together for a final goodbye.

That's when intentional living comes in once again. We can drift off into the sunset or leave with purpose and meaning. There are practical things we can do, like putting financial affairs in order and explaining them to those who need to know. That's a way to prepare loved ones to go on without us, even before they realize what is in their future.

And there are relational things we can do. Saying our goodbyes is emotionally important both for us and our peace as well as the peace of others. At one point in my cancer journey when circumstances looked dire, my adult children gathered. I asked them, "Is there anything you would like to hear me say to you?" One responded that she wanted to know if I was proud of her. I can assure you, since then, I have intentionally said the words, "I'm so proud of you," at every available opportunity.

But sometimes, we can't wrap up loose ends in relationships neatly. The other person has their own free will and may not want to reconcile. I really appreciate the freedom and wisdom of the Bible verse, Romans 12:18, "If possible, so far as it depends on you, be at peace with all men." [18] We can't control how others respond, but we can do what is reasonably possible on our end to make amends.

A few days ago, I was laughing at myself about the little things I have done for my husband and children without them even realizing it — like labeling shelves so that they can find items, throwing away old papers, and helping my husband laugh at some of his annoying habits so he won't be surprised when others struggle with them.

But we've also had serious conversations about memorial services and burial places. We try to approach those conversations in light-hearted ways, almost like it's a celebration that we can still talk about them. Any information I can leave for him about how I want to be remembered will be helpful in the midst of his grief when the time comes.

When Things Are in Order

The more you get off your mind and heart before those final days, I believe the more you will experience peace. My friend Lois wrote me about her brother with terminal cancer, "David and his son, Matt, closed his cabin for the winter. It is difficult to realize that he is not hunting or fishing this winter. Then this morning, he spent some time with our 95-year-old mother and our two sisters. He apologized to Betty for the way he treated her growing up. She was so moved by his sincere apology after all these years."

It's like packing for a trip, thinking about where you are going, and making preparations. The longer you have, the more details you can think through and redesign the plan as circumstances change.

And when the packing is over, and your list runs out, there is peace — peace that what you wanted to get done is finally done, peace that you have done what you could, peace that you are ready for whatever tomorrow will bring. Not everything may be perfect, but you can rest assured that others can and will continue without you.

Kara Tippets blogged throughout her battle with cancer. Towards the end, in her fatigue, she posted this conversation with her husband:

"I once had so much more (energy) to spend, didn't I?"

His gentle answer was, "Yes, dear, but what you had to spend today, you spent well in love." [19]

Although Kara was weak, she was strong. That is how I want my end to be. I can't control what it will look like, but I desire others to see that I lived the time I had making intentional choices of love.

Reflection:

- This chapter has been hard to write and may have been difficult for you to read. What were the most challenging parts for you?

- When you think about those challenging parts, what can you do now to have peace?

It Comes[20]

For some it comes through pain
Years of dying day by day
Wrenching, fighting, coping
With suffering and life's decay.

For others it comes quickly
Stabbing a heart
Unlocking a seat belt
Light slips into darkness

Some face it unjustly
Fiery furnace, a lion's jaw
Blasting guns, roadside bombs
Planes fall from the sky

But for all of us it comes
There is no escaping
We don't choose the means
Only the response, before and after

What we all look for
What we sincerely desire
Is peace.

Maggie Bruehl, 2013
Splash: Captured Moments in Time

For Caregivers

I couldn't end this book without talking with caregivers who have been reading it, either with their loved ones or alone. You have one of the most challenging jobs in all the world, yet you do it with grace and kindness even while grieving the loss you currently have and the loneliness you someday will experience. The ones who have it the hardest are those who read this alone.

It's hard enough to care for another person, but it's even harder to care for someone in denial, who thinks they will get better, this illness has just been a bad dream, or they just close their eyes, shutting out not only the disease but everything that is good around them. It's difficult to reason with someone who won't agree to take their medication or insists on walking when they are no longer able. And it's next to impossible to help someone who wants to control everything around them, including you, their caregiver, because they cannot prevent their physical decline.

If this is you, my heart goes out to you. You are your loved one's lifeline but getting little credit. Few see the sacrifices you make daily of your time and energy.

I want you to know that I see you.

I've been there.

I've done it myself and watched others give their time and energy for what seems to be a thankless job. I've smelled the smells that come with caregiving and held the hand of the dying during their last breaths.

But just you being there with them helps them sense that they are not alone. You give them the dignity of knowing others care.

Their Perspective

Wouldn't it be ideal if your loved one had the balanced perspective talked about in this book, accepting that they have a life-threatening disease and patiently waiting for the end to come? Wouldn't it be wonderful if they recognized the loving things you do for them so that they are not alone?

But we don't live in an ideal world, and for whatever reason, your loved one might not be there. Part of your caregiving job is to help them recognize their journey by speaking lovingly but directly to them about the realities facing them. This book's purpose is to help people gently lean into my journey and identify with the similarities, coming to some of the same conclusions, or at least defining the differences and communicating them to others.

It doesn't help to argue with them. They will push you away, resenting what they may feel is your control when they lack control. The best approach is reasoning with them through a loving relationship. If they can't seem to reason through it, ask yourself what the issue might be: cognitive, emotional, or both. If it is cognitive, simplify the language and try to find ways to communicate so that they will not feel you are talking down to them or have any other motive than their best interest.

My husband's mother had dementia in her last days, and she was fearful of any change. Even getting dressed in the morning made her fearful of where we were going to take her. After a time, our best answer was that we were helping her get ready because she would see her parents soon. Since we believed in heaven, this was enough truth for us, and we communicated it in a way that comforted her.

If a loved one is in denial because of emotional reasons, talking is again the best approach. Explore their past rather than their current condition. You may discover clues that could help you understand what keeps them from accepting their diagnosis. Go with them on appointments so that you know clearly what the doctor has or has not said. A written copy of instructions also helps. If other friends or family reinforce the reality, they may go with what the majority says, but it can also backfire if they become paranoid and think there is a conspiracy against them. One indirect approach I have found helpful is to talk about how other people handle their disease, modeling for my loved one how to live with grace and without fear.

And please don't underestimate how hard it may be for them to depend on you. Most of the pushback is due to their lack of control and embarrassment. They may be depressed, which is hard when you want to hold on to good memories. Try to be encouraging, praising them for what they can do or how they are helping so they feel they have some control in their care. You cannot praise too often; just as you are needy of their praise, they need yours.

Lindsay, an Oncology RN, confessed in her article, "To Every Cancer Patient I Ever Took Care of, I'm Sorry, I Didn't Get It." She explained that among other things she didn't understand as a caregiver, "I didn't get how hard the waiting is. It's literally the worst part." [21]

Your Perspective

Of course, it's hard to work on their perspective if you haven't accepted what the future looks like for your loved one. The best thing for both of you is to educate yourself on their disease. It can help you embrace realistic expectations and plan for your physical, emotional, and financial future as you understand what lies ahead. Realistic expectations give objectivity that is otherwise hard to find and keeps surprises to a minimum.

Emotions may be more difficult to corral. You have the challenge of dealing with your loved one's feelings while dealing with your own, on top of the emotions of others in your life. While your loved one can peacefully slip into a zone, you are left representing them to a world that cares about them and you, or at least is curious. Stretched already with a full life, you have chosen to take on more responsibility for someone you love.

Dick Peterson, a friend who has been caring for his wife with multiple sclerosis for more than 20 years, wrote about the daily realities of caregiving, "Uninvited and unwelcomed, this disease now forces us into a kind of sick reality game, leaving no choice but to follow the rules even as they change and become more restrictive." [22]

And about their future, he projects, "It seems like the sickbed and wheelchair seldom release prisoners. Sleep-deprived nights and need-serving days expect some sort of recompense if only nothing more than evidence of recovery. But a disease that will never be cured and gets worse offers none."

The Good News

The good news is that you do not have to take this on by yourself. During their lifetime, your loved one has hopefully developed a circle of relationships, a community that may be willing to help. As much as you might want to do it all, you can call on them to help. It may be friends from their job, church, hobby group, neighborhood, or professional organization. Often these friends want to lean in but don't know how. As you get to know them and communicate specific needs, they can see ways to help their special friend. Sometimes your friends might want to pitch in to provide for you with needs in your own household.

The key is to ask. People don't know there is a need or that you are open to accepting help unless you communicate it. Others may see you stressed with so many responsibilities, not knowing how or when to jump in to help. Or they may see you as so competent that you don't need any help. Be honest with ourselves and others about our limitations and when a break would be welcomed. We need to pace our focus and energy to have reserves for when things do hit those hard days.

CaringBridge.com is a tool I have found helpful in caring for others as well as helping my family care for me. It allows you to communicate online with a broad scope of people instead of talking with everyone individually. It's easy to set up and manage, adding journal entries as time progresses. I let family and friends know about the site, encouraging them to set up email notifications for when there is an update. CaringBridge also has a response mechanism for friends and long-distance relatives to communicate their love and support. You can use websites to schedule meals, coordinate visitation, and post pictures to share with others. Who doesn't love a picture to spark a memory and conversation?

A couple of years ago, my friend Nancy came to the end of her life. Since she was a traveling missionary, she had friends and contacts worldwide. While she wanted to be with each one, her strength was failing. We arranged for her to text me whatever she wanted to say to them, and I would post it on CaringBridge so they could hear her heart. I even ghost-wrote for her (with her permission) as she became weaker since I knew her perspective towards her death and what she would want to say. After she died, I passed on Memorial Service information with internet links so that people from Africa, Europe, and Asia could join. And afterward, I corresponded with some of her friends through their grief.

But I also recognize that sometimes, there is a lack of a natural community. That's when you can lean into medical and community resources. I've found doctor's offices and hospitals very helpful, some even having social workers who have connections with agencies and financial resources. For example, my local cancer center has support groups for patients as well as caregivers. They realize the value you bring and the importance of taking care of yourself so that you can care for others.

There are also financial services you can contact online like www.socialsecurity.gov, www.va.gov, www.copays.org, www.healthwellfoundation.org, and www.needymeds.org for financial assistance. Some resources are specific to the disease, like www.cancercare.org and www.cancerfac.org. Others can connect you with caregivers going through similar challenges for emotional support (an example: https://www.asbestos.com/blog/2023/04/10/mesothelioma-caregivers-support-community/).

When the time comes, government aid provides hospice care

and similar agencies. I recommend hospice to everyone as a medical, emotional, physical, and spiritual resource. Ask your doctor when you think your loved one is physically ready for this stage. I've known people who have been able to use these resources for months rather than weeks before their loved ones passed. These angels know the difficulty of this time in your life and want to be by your side as you consider what is best for your loved one.

My son-in-law Jason initially refused to accept hospice. To him, it was like admitting defeat, that he couldn't kick his leukemia. While I was driving him home from a doctor's appointment, I explained to him that the benefits of hospice were not only for him but for his family, providing assistance and emotional support when he could not. When the focus was turned from hospice helping him to hospice to helping his family, his heart was touched. It was an extra benefit to him when he realized he could do his transfusions at the hospice center, sharing a room with an outdoor patio with his wife so they could watch the birds! If every caregiver knew of the resources available and took full advantage of them, their job might be easier.

One last thought, please take care of yourself as a caregiver. If you are run down, anxious, or irritated, your loved one can sense it. Be brave enough to ask family and friends to relieve you. Take time off and refresh yourself as needed. We need you for the long haul, so pace yourself and your needs.

For all of us living with a disease that will likely take our lives, thank you for all you do as a caregiver to make us comfortable. Thank you for reflecting the truth to us when it is hard to accept. Thank you for the appointments you have made, canceled, and then made again. Thank you for the wheelchairs you have maneuvered and the medicine boxes you have filled. Thank you for the messes you have cleaned and the patience you have shown. Thank you for your kindness when we have been less than kind. Thank you for the endless hours you have read to us, held our hand, and prayed over us.

Most of all, thank you for your sacrifice of love.

Reflection:

- What emotions do you bring with you to the job of caregiving? What in the chapter encourages you the most?

- Where can you get help with your caretaking duties? What can you do today to take care of yourself?

In Case You Are Interested

You may have wondered what gave me the perspective in this book as well as strength on those dark days when I couldn't lift my head. How did I power through sixteen years of cancer, seven broken bones, a hip replacement, and a bone marrow transplant?

The most important factor in my journey has been my relationship with God through Jesus Christ. The philosopher Pascal is credited with saying, "There is a God-shaped vacuum in the heart of each man which cannot be satisfied by any created thing but only by God the Creator, made known through Jesus Christ." [23]

Religion is a set of rules that, if you believe hard enough or are good enough, someday connect you with God. Jesus offers an alternative, suggesting that God desires a relationship with us, joining the Jewish Old Testament promise of a Messiah with Jesus' claim to be the Son of God. The simplest way I can explain how to have this relationship with God is through the "Four Spiritual Laws." [24] I was trying to fill the emptiness Pascal described with other things when a friend shared these four principles with me.

The intro said, "Just as there are physical laws that govern the physical universe, so there are spiritual laws that govern your relationship with God." It made sense to me that there are scientific truths that govern the universe. I didn't disagree with evolution and yet was mystified by the beauty around me that went beyond survival of the fittest.

The first point, "God loves you and has a wonderful plan for your life," really caught my attention, including Bible verses describing God's love. I had never thought about a personal, emotional God who had desires towards me — it had always been my search for God. I had never thought of God having a purpose or plan for my life, but that also made sense. If there was a God powerful enough to create me and put me on this earth, then he certainly had a plan for my direction.

The second point explained why I wasn't experiencing the connection with God: "Man is sinful and separated from God. Therefore, he cannot know and experience God's love and plan for his life." It described sin as "self-will, characterized by an attitude of active rebellion or passive indifference." This was new to me because I thought sin was an action, like doing something evil, not an attitude. But I could understand how my attitude *towards* God was separating me *from* God.

The third point was: "Jesus Christ is God's only provision for man's sin. Through Him, you can know and experience God's love and plan for your life." In my personal study of religion, none of the religious leaders I read about claimed to be the "Son of God" like Jesus did. They did not offer to bridge our attitude of sin with God's perfection. Either Jesus was who he said he was, or, as C.S. Lewis put it, "A man who was merely a man and said the sort of things Jesus said would not be a great moral teacher. He would either be a lunatic on the level with the man who says he is a poached egg, or else he would be the Devil of Hell. You must make your choice."[25]

How do we make a choice? The fourth point said, "We must individually receive Jesus Christ as Savior and Lord; then we can know and experience God's love and plan for our lives." That made sense — if it was my attitude leading to actions that separated me, then believing in Jesus was the key. I could never do enough good deeds and desired a relationship on God's terms.

Having a personal relationship with God through Jesus has made all the difference in my life. Instead of the Bible being just a good book, now it's a love letter from him to me. I've also felt God's peace and presence in the hard times when I was suffering or close to death. It's given me a community of believers who, although not perfect, are the most loving, caring people I know.

In earlier chapters, we talked about how faith is important on our

IN CASE YOU ARE INTERESTED

journey, and I challenged you, "If your current belief system does not give you hope and peace, you might want to find one that does."

I want to repeat that challenge and ask you to consider trusting Jesus.

Reflection:

- Where are you on your spiritual journey? What do you believe about Jesus and his claims?

- Are you ready to trust Jesus with your life? If so, simply talk to god and tell him in your own words.

- If you would like to contact me, email Maggie.bruehl@gmail.com.

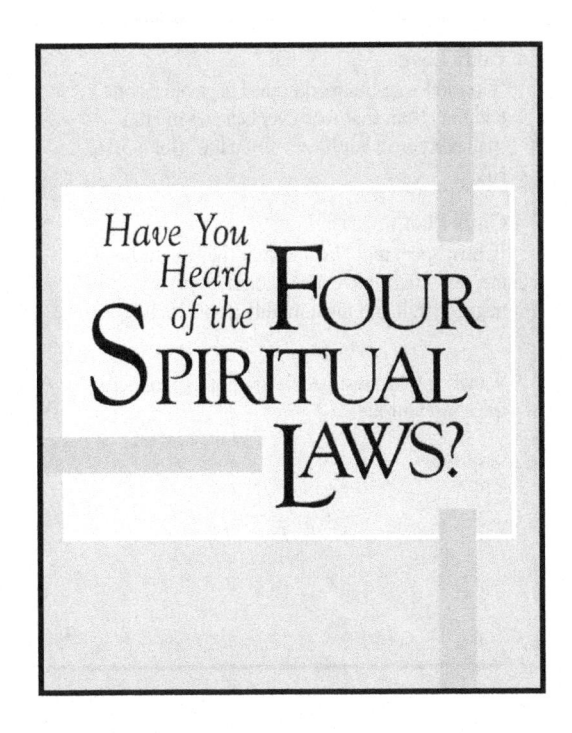

Have You Heard of the **FOUR SPIRITUAL LAWS?**

Just as there are physical laws
that govern the physical universe,
so are there spiritual laws that govern
your relationship with God.

LAW 1

*God **loves** you and offers a wonderful **plan** for your life.*

(References contained in this booklet should be read in context from the Bible wherever possible.)

2

God's Love
"God so loved the world that He gave His one and only Son, that who ever believes in Him shall not perish but have eternal life" (John 3:16, NIV).

God's Plan
[Christ speaking] "I came that they might have life, and might have it abundantly" [that it might be full and meaningful] (John 10:10).

Why is it that most people are not experiencing the abundant life?

Because...

3

LAW 2

*Man is **sinful** and **separated** from God. Therefore, he cannot know and experience God's love and plan for his life.*

Man Is Sinful
"All have sinned and fall short of the glory of God" (Romans 3:23).

Man was created to have fellowship with God; but, because of his own stubborn self-will, he chose to go his own independent way and fellowship with God was broken. This self-will, characterized by an attitude of active rebellion or passive indifference, is an evidence of what the Bible calls sin.

4

Man Is Separated
"The wages of sin is death" [spiritual separation from God] (Romans 6:23).

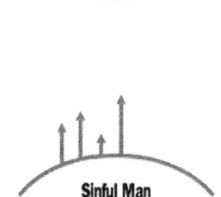

This diagram illustrates that God is holy and man is sinful. A great gulf separates the two. The arrows illustrate that man is continually trying to reach God and the abundant life through his own efforts, such as a good life, philosophy, or religion—but he inevitably fails.

The third law explains the only way to bridge this gulf...

5

LAW 3

*Jesus Christ is God's **only** provision for man's sin. Through Him you can know and experience God's love and plan for your life.*

He Died In Our Place
"God demonstrates His own love toward us, in that while we were yet sinners, Christ died for us" (Romans 5:8).

He Rose from the Dead
"Christ died for our sins...He was buried...He was raised on the third day, according to the Scriptures...He appeared to Peter, then to the twelve. After that He appeared to more than five hundred..." (1 Corinthians 15:3-6).

6

He Is the Only Way to God
"Jesus said to him, 'I am the way, and the truth, and the life; no one comes to the Father but through Me'" (John 14:6).

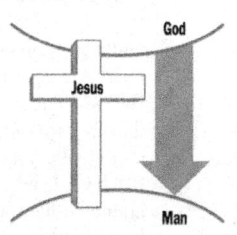

God
Jesus
Man

This diagram illustrates that God has bridged the gulf that separates us from Him by sending His Son, Jesus Christ, to die on the cross in our place to pay the penalty for our sins.

It is not enough just to know these three laws...

7

LAW 4

We must individually receive Jesus Christ as Savior and Lord; then we can know and experience God's love and plan for our lives.

We Must Receive Christ
"As many as received Him, to them He gave the right to become children of God, even to those who believe in His name" (John 1:12).

We Receive Christ Through Faith
"By grace you have been saved through faith; and that not of yourselves, it is the gift of God; not as a result of works that no one should boast" (Ephesians 2:8,9).

When We Receive Christ, We Experience a New Birth
(Read John 3:1–8.)

8

We Receive Christ Through Personal Invitation
[Christ speaking] "Behold, I stand at the door and knock; if any one hears My voice and opens the door, I will come in to him" (Revelation 3:20).

Receiving Christ involves turning to God from self (repentance) and trusting Christ to come into our lives to forgive our sins and to make us what He wants us to be. Just to agree **intellectually** that Jesus Christ is the Son of God and that He died on the cross for our sins is not enough. Nor is it enough to have an **emotional** experience. We receive Jesus Christ by **faith**, as an act of the **will**.

These two circles represent two kinds of lives:

Self-Directed Life
S - Self is on the throne
† - Christ is outside the life
● - Interests are directed by self, often resulting in discord and frustration

Christ-Directed Life
† - Christ is in the life and on the throne
S - Self is yielding to Christ
● - Interests are directed by Christ, resulting in harmony with God's plan

Which circle best represents your life?
Which circle would you like to have represent your life?

9

The following explains how you can receive Christ:

You Can Receive Christ Right Now by Faith Through Prayer
(Prayer is talking with God)
God knows your heart and is not so concerned with your words as He is with the attitude of your heart. The following is a suggested prayer:

> Lord Jesus, I need You. Thank You for dying on the cross for my sins. I open the door of my life and receive You as my Savior and Lord. Thank You for forgiving my sins and giving me eternal life. Take control of the throne of my life. Make me the kind of person You want me to be.

Does this prayer express the desire of your heart?

If it does, I invite you to pray this prayer right now, and Christ will come into your life, as He promised.

10

How to Know That Christ Is in Your Life
Did you receive Christ into your life? According to His promise in Revelation 3:20, where is Christ right now in relation to you? Christ said He would come into your life. Would He mislead you? On what authority do you know God has answered your prayer? (The trustworthiness of God Himself and His Word.)

The Bible Promises Eternal Life to All Who Receive Christ
"God has given us eternal life, and this life is in His Son. He who has the Son has the life; he who does not have the Son of God does not have the life. These things I have written to you who believe in the name of the Son of God, in order that you may **know** that you have eternal life" (1 John 5:11–13).

Thank God often that Christ is in your life and that He will never leave you (Hebrews 13:5). You can know on the basis of His promise that Christ lives in you and that you have eternal life from the very moment you invite Him in. He will not deceive you.

11

FINISHING STRONG

An important reminder...

Do Not Depend on Feelings
The promise of God's Word, the Bible—not our feelings—is our authority. The Christian lives by faith (trust) in the trustworthiness of God Himself and His Word. This train diagram illustrates the relationship among **fact** (God and His Word), **faith** (our trust in God and His Word), and **feeling** (the result of our faith and obedience). (Read John 14:21.)

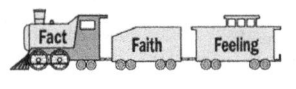

The train will run with or without the caboose. However, it would be useless to attempt to pull the train by the caboose. In the same way, as Christians we do not depend on feelings or emotions, but we place our faith (trust) in the trustworthiness of God and the promises of His Word.

Now That You Have Received Christ
The moment you received Christ by faith, as an act of the will, many things happened, including the following:

- Christ came into your life (Revelation 3:20; Colossians 1:27).
- Your sins were forgiven (Colossians 1:14).
- You became a child of God (John 1:12).
- You received eternal life (John 5:24).
- You began the great adventure for which God created you (John 10:10; 2 Corinthians 5:17; 1 Thessalonians 5:18).

Can you think of anything more wonderful that could happen to you than receiving Christ? Would you like to thank God in prayer right now for what He has done for you? By thanking God, you demonstrate your faith.

To enjoy your new life to the fullest...

Suggestions for Christian Growth
Spiritual growth results from trusting Jesus Christ. "The righteous man shall live by faith" (Galatians 3:11). A life of faith will enable you to trust God increasingly with every detail of your life, and to practice the following:

- **G** *Go* to God in prayer daily (John 15:7).
- **R** *Read* God's Word daily (Acts 17:11); begin with the Gospel of John.
- **O** *Obey* God moment by moment (John 14:21).
- **W** *Witness* for Christ by your life and words (Matthew 4:19; John 15:8).
- **T** *Trust* God for every detail of your life (1 Peter 5:7).
- **H** *Holy Spirit*—allow Him to control and empower your daily life and witness (Galatians 5:16,17; Acts 1:8).

Fellowship in a Good Church
God's Word instructs us not to forsake "the assembling of ourselves together" (Hebrews 10:25). Several logs burn brightly together, but put one aside on the cold hearth and the fire goes out. So it is with your relationship with other Christians.

If you do not belong to a church, do not wait to be invited. Take the initiative; call the pastor of a nearby church where Christ is honored and His Word is preached. Start this week, and make plans to attend regularly.

Special Materials Are Available for Christian Growth
If you have come to know Christ personally through this presentation of the gospel or would like further help in getting to know Christ better, two sites are recommended:
www.startingwithGod.com or www.growinginChrist.com

If you still have questions, visit:
www.whoisJesus-really.com or www.everystudent.com

If this booklet has been helpful to you, please share it with someone else.

To encourage the widest distribution possible, this booklet is available at a nominal price for use by you or your organization. You may place your name or the name of your organization in the space below.

ISBN 1-56399-019-9

CAMPUS CRUSADE FOR CHRIST

Written by Bill Bright. Copyright 2007 Bright Media Foundation and Campus Crusade for Christ. Formerly Copyright 1965-2006 Campus Crusade for Christ, Inc. All rights reserved. No part of this booklet may be changed in any way or reproduced in any form without written permission from Campus Crusade for Christ. Published by Campus Crusade for Christ, 375 Highway 74 South, Suite A, Peachtree City, GA 30269. Printed in the United States of America. www.campuscrusade.org

Acknowledgments

So many people have helped me along the journey of this book as I wrote and rewrote, as health permitted. Friends and family, too extensive to mention, have been with me every step of the way, patient with my frustrated dreams. I hope they know how deeply they are appreciated.

I especially want to thank Nancy Beverly for being my "coach" and rough draft editor, holding me responsible for the dates and goals I set. Word Weavers International was my source of encouragement and editing, especially in the latest version, as I struggled with a final direction.

And I appreciate those who contributed stories, personally or through their blogs, giving me strength and affirmation. Blogs tend to be more real and vulnerable than books and articles as authors process their reflections and emotions in the present tense. I've walked alongside them and wept for them when they left us.

Most importantly, I acknowledge my husband, Roger, for his endless patience and encouragement. What would I do without you?

I hope I never have to answer that question.

Resources

Suggested Resources

- *Splash: Captured Moments in Time* is a book of poetry I wrote several years ago. The last section, Splash of a Boulder, is a collection of poems from my cancer journey.

- Kara Tippets was a Christian blogger I followed for years who had a way of drawing you into her story, even if you were not experiencing a life-threatening illness. Her writing was edited, and she is credited with writing:

    o The Hardest Peace: Expecting Grace in the Midst of Life's Hard

    o Just Show Up: The Dance of Walking through Suffering Together

    o And It Was Beautiful: Celebrating Life in the Midst of the Long Good-Bye

    o Big Love: the practice of loving beyond your limits

    o The Long Goodbye: The Kara Tippett's Story (also a streaming movie by this title)

- James E. Miller's **When You Know You're Dying: 12 Thoughts to Guide you Through the Days Ahead** (Willowgreen Publishing, 1997) is a short 61-page booklet that echoes many of the thoughts communicated throughout this book. They are in a bullet point format that makes the book a quick and easy read.

- For Christians or those who want more information from the Bible concerning suffering and the end of life, Kelly Mize wrote, **Preparing for Metamorphosis: Life after the Worst Diagnosis** (Blue Sky Daisies, 2022, Wichita, KS). She is no longer with us but had a perspective, including scripture verses, that gave her peace towards the end of her life.

- Also from a Christian perspective, **Strength for the Cancer Journey** (Moody Publishers, 2020) by Deborah Barr is a cross between a devotional and a journal in hardcover, which makes it a nice gift.

Endnotes

1. Maggie Bruehl, Splash: **Defining Moments in Time**, (Bloomington, IN: WestBow Press, 2013) 102-103.

2. American Society of Clinical Oncology, https://www.asco.org

3. John Smith, http://goodbloodbadblood.worpress.com/2014/07/08/the-university-of-cancer-part-2/

4. Tim Keller, https://www.theatlantic.com/ideas/archive/2021/03/tim-keller-growing-my-faith-face-death/618219/

5. Kara Tippets – https://www.mundanefaithfulness.com/home/tag/Blog

6. Romans 8:28, **The New American Standard Bible** (La Habra, CA: Lockman Foundation, 2020).

7. Robert Carr, https://howtoliveameaningfullife.com/do-we-have-any-control-over-our-fate/

8. Used with permission; names have been changed.

9. Terry Morgan, https://maturitascafe.com, used with permission.

10 Kate Bowler, http://www.nytimes.com/2016/02/14/opinion/sunday/death-the-prosperity-gospel-and-me.html?smprod=nytcore-ipone&smid=nytcore-iphone-share

11 Tim Keller, https://www.theatlantic.com/ideas/archive/2021/03/tim-keller-growing-my-faith-face-death/618219/

12 Recognizing Milestones, http://www.cancer.net/surviorship/life-after-cancer/recognizing-milestones

13 The Fruit of Leukemia: Life-Changing Perspectives, by Cancerwise Blogger on August 22, 2012, http://www2.mdanderson.org/cancerwise/2012/08-the-fruit-of-leukemia-life-changing-perspectives.html

14 Oliver Sacks, https://www.nytimes.com/2015/02/19/opinion/oliver-sacks-on-learning-he-has-terminal-cancer.html

15 Ethan Remmel, (deceased) https://www.psychologytoday.com/us/blog/living-while-dying/201104/the-meaning-suffering

16 Laurie Beckland, https://www.naaccr.org/as-i-lay-dying/

17 Ethan Remmel, (deceased) https://www.psychologytoday.com/us/blog/living-while-dying/201104/the-meaning-suffering

18 Romans 12:18, **New American Standard Bible**, 1995, Lockman Foundation, LaHabra, CA.

19 Kara Tippets, https://www.mundanefaithfulness.com/home/tag/Blog

20 Maggie Bruehl, Splash: **Defining Moments in Time**, (Bloomington, IN: WestBow Press, 2013) 97.

21 Lindsay Norris, https://www.huffpost.com/entry/dear-every-cancer-patient-i-ever-took-care-of-im_b_58348345e4b050dfe61876d7.

22 More of Dick's perspective as a caregiver is contained in "Living with and Intruder," https://www.todayschristianwoman.com/articles/2008/september/livingintruder.html

23 Pascal, https://www.goodreads.com/quotes/801132-there-is-a-god-shaped-vacuum-in-the-heart-of-each#:~:text=Learn%20more),"There%20is%20a%20God%2Dshaped%20vacuum%20in%20the%20heart%20of,made%20know%20through%20Jesus%20Christ."

24 Used with permission, https://campusministry.org/docs/tools/FourSpiritualLaws.pdf.

25 CS Lewis, Mere Christianity, https://en.wikipedia.org/wiki/Lewis%27s_trilemma#:~:text=A%20man%20who%20was%20merely,You%20must%20make%20your%20choice.

Other conversations or correspondence used
with permission. In some cases, names have been
changed to protect privacy.

Made in the USA
Columbia, SC
02 December 2023